MAY 2001

ENVIRONMENTAL HEALTH COMPETENCY PROJECT

Recommendations for Core

Competencies for Local

Environmental Health

Practitioners

National Center for Environmental Health, Centers for Disease Control and Prevention
American Public Health Association

Revised June 27, 2001

ENVIRONMENTAL HEALTH
COMPETENCY PROJECT:
Recommendations
for Core Competencies
for Local Environmental Health Practitioners

American Public Health Association

National Center for Environmental Health,
Centers for Disease Control and Prevention
May 2001

Revised June 27, 2001

ACKNOWLEDGEMENTS

We are grateful to the numerous organizations and agencies that provided information from the field and contributing to the development of this report. These individuals contributed a considerable amount of time and energy to the project.

In addition to the organizations mentioned in the report, we'd like to thank Dr. Thomas A. Burke, Larry Gordon, and Petrona Lee for their inspiration and contributions. We would like to express deep gratitude to the staff of the organizations who provided support. Special thanks are given to Annette Ferebee, Julie Desai, Heidi Klein, and Gilah Langner.

This project would not have been possible without the support of the National Center for Environmental Health at the Centers for Disease Control and Prevention. We especially want to acknowledge the work of Patrick Bohan, RS, MS, MSEH whose foresight made this project a reality.

For additional information about this project, please email EHSB@cdc.gov.

Revised June 27, 2001

Table of Contents

Revised June 27, 2001

EXECUTIVE SUMMARY

In February 2000, environmental health experts from 13 national environmental/health organizations came together in Washington to begin the work of defining core competencies for local level environmental health practitioners. APHA's Public Health Innovations Project, with funding from the National Center for Environmental Health (NCEH) at the Centers for Disease Control and Prevention (CDC), convened the meeting.

The expert panel members and several federal agency representatives met for two days to identify the core competencies local environmental health practitioners needed to be effective in their work. The following 14 core competencies reflect the outcome of that meeting. The competencies are grouped into the three primary functions of an environmental health program – assessment, management and communication.

A. ASSESSMENT

- **Information Gathering**: The capacity to identify sources and compile relevant and appropriate information when needed, and the knowledge of where to go to obtain the information.
- **Data Analysis and Interpretation**: The capacity to analyze data, recognize meaningful test results, interpret results, and present the results in an appropriate way to different types of audiences.
- **Evaluation**: The capacity to evaluate the effectiveness or performance of procedures, interventions, and programs.

B. MANAGEMENT

- **Problem Solving**: The capacity to develop insight into and appropriate solutions to environmental health problems.
- **Economic and Political Issues**: The capacity to understand and appropriately utilize information concerning the economic and political implications of decisions.
- **Organizational Knowledge and Behavior**: The capacity to function effectively within the culture of the organization and to be an effective team player.
- **Project Management**: The capacity to plan, implement, and maintain fiscally responsible programs/projects using appropriate skills, and prioritize projects across the employee's entire workload.
- **Computer & Information Technology**: The capacity to utilize information technology as needed to produce work products.
- **Reporting, Documentation, and Record-Keeping**: The capacity to produce reports to document actions, keep records, and inform appropriate parties.
- **Collaboration**: The capacity to form partnerships and alliances with other individuals and organizations in order to enhance performance on the job.

C. COMMUNICATION

- **Educate:** The capacity to use the environmental health practitioner's front-line role to effectively educate the public on environmental health issues and the public health rationale for recommendations.
- **Communicate:** The capacity to effectively communicate risk and exchange information with colleagues, other practitioners, clients, policy-makers, interest groups, media, and the public through routine activities, public speaking, print and electronic media, and interpersonal relations.
- **Conflict Resolution:** The capacity to facilitate the resolution of conflicts within the agency, in the community, and with regulated parties.
- **Marketing:** The capacity to articulate basic concepts of environmental health and public health and convey an understanding of their value and importance to clients and the public.

Identifying these core competencies is just the first step. They are viewed as a "work in progress" and feedback from the field is welcome.

PART I: **SETTING THE STAGE**

A.   **INTRODUCTION**

The goal of this project is to provide broadly accepted guidelines and recommendations to local public health leaders for the core competencies needed by local environmental health practitioners working in local health departments (LHDs) to strengthen their capacities to anticipate, recognize, and respond to environmental health challenges.

This report is based on a meeting, held February 28 through March 1, 2000, in Washington, D.C., and on subsequent discussions with partner organizations and representatives. The meeting was convened to build on existing work in the field of environmental health competencies and to outline the core competencies needed to effectively carry out environmental health programs at the local level. These competencies complement the technical competencies developed by the National Environmental Health Association (NEHA) and are considered necessary regardless of the setting---rural or urban---for environmental health practitioners in LHDs.

Environmental health is a key component of public health. Local environmental health practitioners are the "front-line troops" in the public health battle to prevent disease. Yet many people working in LHDs have no formal training in environmental health or public health. By attempting to identify the core competencies necessary for effective environmental health at the local level and beginning to develop consensus on their acceptance, we can strengthen the environmental health infrastructure and build the capacity of local programs.

> **Environmental Health and Protection**
>
> Environmental health and protection is the art and science of protecting against environmental factors that adversely impact human health or the ecologic balances to long-term human health and environmental quality, whether in the natural or human-made environment. These factors include, but are not limited to air, food and water contaminants; radiation, toxic chemicals, wastes, disease vectors, safety hazards, and habitat alterations. (*The Future of Environmental Health,* JEH, Vol. 55, No. 4, 28-32, 1993)

B. Background

Sponsored by the American Public Health Association (APHA) and the National Center for Environmental Health (NCEH) of the Centers for Disease Control and Prevention (CDC), the Environmental Health Competency Project convened an Expert Panel, comprising a wide variety of environmental and public health associations and organizations.   The 13 panelists (Appendix A) represent the following national organizations: The American Academy of Sanitarians (AAS), the Association of Environmental Health Academic Programs (AEHAP), the Association of Public Health Laboratories (APHL), the Association of Schools of Public Health (ASPH), the Association of State and Territorial Health Officials (ASTHO), the Council of State and Territorial Epidemiologists (CSTE), the International Association for Food Protection (IAFP), the National Association of County and City Health Officials (NACCHO), the National Association of Local Boards of Health (NALBOH), the National Conference of Local Environmental Health Administrators (NCLEHA), the National Rural Health Association (NRHA) and NEHA. Participating federal agencies included the Agency for Toxic Substances and Disease Registry (ATSDR), the U.S. Department of Agriculture's Food Safety and Inspection Services (USDA), the U.S. Environmental Protection Agency (EPA), the Food and Drug Administration (FDA), and the Health Resources and Services Administration (HRSA).

Before the meeting, members of the Expert Panel responded to a short questionnaire about competencies. The facilitator used these responses to gain an understanding of panelists' opinions about potential competencies, identify areas of agreement and disagreement among panelists, and focus meeting activities. The goal of the meeting was to provide the foundation for a preliminary list of core competencies for local environmental health practitioners and to delineate areas of consensus among Expert Panelists. The panelists were then encouraged to take the recommendations report back to their affiliated organizations and begin assessing, modifying, and encouraging support for the competencies. A summary of the Expert Panel discussion is located in Appendix B.

The Environmental Health Competency Project contributes to the development of an overall public health infrastructure, in concert with other programs now being implemented, such as the Healthy People 2010 Infrastructure Initiative, the National Public Health Performance Standards Program, and the Public Health Workforce 21st Century Agenda. All of these efforts are laying important groundwork to help move the public health community toward greater excellence in public health practice.

C. Definitions

The target audience for these recommendations is environmental health practitioners who work in LHDs. For this project, an **environmental health practitioner** is defined as a person working in an environmental health position in a LHD who has at least an undergraduate degree with one to four years of experience.

A LHD is defined as a statutorily designated agency of local government charged with delivering identifiable health services designed to prevent or solve public health problems. Nearly 3,000 LHDs, as defined above, exist in the United States. Most have a broad range of environmental health responsibilities, including food safety, drinking water safety, solid and liquid waste disposal, hazardous waste disposal, vector control, and institutional health. (See Appendix C)

A primary objective of environmental health programs is to prevent death and illness from environmentally related disease and injury. The ability to anticipate, recognize, and respond to environmental health threats is necessary to achieve this objective. Recent widely publicized outbreaks of illness---caused by Cryptosporidium in the Milwaukee water supply, the emergence of *Escherichia* coli O157:H7 in food, and hantavirus in the rodent population---only underscore the need for environmental health programs that are adequately staffed and capable of anticipating and responding quickly and with flexibility to environmental health threats. This includes addressing emerging environmentally related public health problems.

> *There is a strong need to prepare the environmental health workforce to address the complex environmental health problems facing the nation in the 21st century.*

Although this report is targeted to LHDs, the panel recognizes that many people work in environmental health positions in agencies other than local public health. The competencies developed in this report may apply to these people.

D. Definition of Competencies

For this project, the panel defined a competency as:

> **a cluster of related knowledge, skills, and attitudes that affect a major part of one's job (a role or responsibility), that correlates with performance on the job, that can be measured against some accepted standards, and that can be improved via training and development.** (Parry, S.R. "The Quest for Competencies." *Training*, July 1996, p. 50)

This project builds on the extensive groundwork in this field during the past few years. Examples of recent work on competencies include: The Public Health Functions Workgroup Project, sponsored by the U.S. Department of Health and Human Services (DHHS), Competency-Based Curriculum Work Group; The National Public Health

Performance Standards Program, a collaborative effort by NACCHO, NALBOH, ASTHO, PHF, and APHA and CDC; The Crossroads Colloquium: An Examination of the Educational Needs for Environmental Health and Protection; The Public Health Faculty/Agency Forum sponsored by DHHS and CDC; and NEHA's Committee on the Future of Environmental Health.

E. Basic Assumptions

A basic assumption of this project is that environmental health practitioners have the *technical* competency to do their jobs.   NEHA's Registered Environmental Health Specialist/Registered Sanitarian (REHS/RS) exam provides a measure of the technical skills essential for the environmental health practitioner. Appendix D lists the technical competencies covered in NEHA's REHS/RS exam; Appendix E lists the content areas covered.

Among the foundational elements of core competencies, the Expert Panel emphasized the following:

- Environmental health practitioners should understand basic public health principles, and the interdisciplinary nature of environmental health.
- Environmental health practitioners should understand environmental protection and environmental health principles and practices.
- Environmental health practitioners should understand basic government functions.
- Environmental health practitioners should understand and be sensitive to the different cultures found in their institutions and communities.

PART II: RECOMMENDED COMPETENCIES

Fourteen core competencies for environmental health practitioners are presented below, based on the work done by the Expert Panel at its February meeting and by subsequent revisions and incorporated comments by the panel. The competencies are grouped into the three primary functions of an environmental health program.

A. **Assessment**

   Information Gathering

   Data Analysis & Interpretation

   Evaluation

B. **Management**

   Problem Solving

   Economic & Political Issues

   Organizational Knowledge & Behavior

   Project Management

   Computer & Information Technology

   Reporting, Documentation, and Record-Keeping

   Collaboration

C. **Communication**

   Educate

   Communicate

   Conflict Resolution

   Marketing

Note: Discussion was extensive about cultural sensitivity as a competency. All participants thought issues of culture are important to being effective, and although not an explicit competency, cultural sensitivity was considered part of all that is done in environmental health and protection. It includes, but is not limited to: understanding the dynamics of cultural diversity (race, ethnicity, and socio-economics); linking with others disciplines inside and outside the agency to enhance the receptivity of the workplace to a multicultural environment; acting with sensitivity and understanding; and developing and adapting approaches to problems that take into account cultural differences.

A. Assessment

A1. <u>Information Gathering</u>: The capacity to identify sources and compile relevant and appropriate information when needed, and the knowledge of where to go to obtain the information.

Examples:

- Literature search in response to a request for information.
- Consult with experts in the field, such as toxicologists, epidemiologists, forensic specialists, and/or environmental engineers.
- Identify, locate and use appropriate reference material (statutes, regulations, reference books, journals).

A2. <u>Data Analysis and Interpretation</u>: The capacity to analyze data, recognize meaningful test results, interpret results, and present the results in an appropriate way to different types of audiences.

Examples:

- Read and summarize technical papers, understand tabular and graphical presentations of data, and translate them for a non-technical audience, for example, translate data from papers published in academic journals into public information materials.
- Analyze data generated internally using simple statistics (e.g., percentages, averages, medians).
- Understand how statistical surveys are performed and what results mean.
- Communicate results to a variety of audiences, using appropriate media.

A3. <u>Evaluation</u>: The capacity to evaluate the effectiveness or performance of procedures, interventions, and programs.

Examples:

- Evaluate the agency's procedures against a given set of standards, such as state requirements.
- Evaluate the results of particular interventions, such as providing information to a group of restaurant managers to resolve food service problems, and determine what improvements have been made after a specified time.
- Evaluate the overall environmental health program in which the practitioner is

working, in terms of inputs (such as number of inspections, number of hotline calls processed) or outcomes (real-world results, progress).

Note: Solo environmental health practitioners may have more occasions to undertake program evaluations than do practitioners working in larger agencies.

B. Management

B1. <u>Problem Solving</u>: The capacity to develop insight into and appropriate solutions to environmental health problems.

Examples:

- Determine the nature of a problem in broader context by asking appropriate questions and reviewing documentation.
- Clearly articulate problem.
- Take appropriate measures to resolve the problem and/or present a range of solutions.
- Collaborate in decision-making process.

B2. <u>Economic and Political Issues</u>: The capacity to understand and appropriately use information about the economic and political implications of decisions.

Examples:

- Understand and maintain awareness of basic economic issues, for example, in interacting with small business owners and communities.
- Understand local history and community demographics, as well as cultural and political issues and sensitivities.
- Enforce regulations equitably and consistently--but with an awareness of the political realities of the work.
- Develop and present options and recommendations that demonstrate an understanding of economic and political conditions in an effort to find appropriate solutions and prioritize actions.
- Understand the economic and political underpinnings and implications of broader agency priorities/decisions.

B3. __Organizational Knowledge and Behavior__**: The capacity to function effectively within the culture of the organization and to be an effective team player.**

Examples:

- Understand the formal legislative/administrative system within which the agency operates.

- Be aware of internal agency functions, priorities, and dynamics.

- Identify and recognize how agendas are set and pursued and how they affect public health.

- Inform supervisor and other appropriate persons about political issues as they arise.

B4. __Project Management__**: The capacity to plan, implement, and maintain fiscally responsible programs and projects using skills and prioritize projects across the employee's entire workload.**

Examples:

- Formulate goals and objectives. Understand what's necessary to get things done, internally and externally.

- Design action steps using a variety of resources.

- Establish appropriate timelines and deadlines.

- Balance the workload when involved in multiple projects.

- Measure outcomes for the program.

- Understand and work effectively within the constraints of fiscal realities.

- Manage programs within budgetary constraints.

- Prioritize budget decisions.

- Monitor expenditures and revenues.

- Recognize and pursue opportunities for external funding.

- Understand the agency's finance system, including purchase requisitions, purchase orders, unencumbered and encumbered funds, allocations, and budget revision.

B5. <u>Computer/Information Technology</u>: **The capacity to use information technology as needed to produce work products.**

Examples:

- Use software available within the agency to perform research, record keeping, communication (e.g., e-mail, word processing programs), data analysis, and interpretation (including simple spreadsheet programs), and reporting tasks.
- Use Web-based applications, such as searching and retrieving information.

B6. <u>Reporting, Documentation, and Record-Keeping</u>: **The capacity to produce reports to document actions, keep records, and inform appropriate parties.**

Examples:

- Generate an inspection report.
- Produce a periodic (e.g., quarterly) activity report.
- Generate a progress report for a grant.
- Maintain organized, accurate, and up-to-date files and records (electronic and/or hard copy).
- Prepare evidence for court cases.

B7. <u>Collaboration</u>: **The capacity to form partnerships and alliances with other individuals and organizations to enhance performance on the job.**

Examples:

- Identify key persons in organizations, community, and media. Networks can be internal to the agency, (e.g., with epidemiologists; public health nurses, and educators; in-house laboratories; plumbing, electrical, and building inspectors) community-wide, (e.g., with nongovernmental organizations, industry, academia, labs) or within the government's public health/environmental protection system (EPA, CDC, other federal agencies; state offices such as State Engineer, Attorney General; and local agencies).
- Cultivate effective links and partnerships by using communications skills; maintaining regular/periodic contact; participating in practitioner organizations; and providing reciprocal help, service, and support.

C. Communication

C1. <u>Educate</u>: The capacity to use the environmental health practitioner's front-line role to effectively educate the public on environmental health issues and the public health rationale for recommendations.

Examples:

- Identify "teaching moments" as part of regulatory function, and opportunities to share "lessons learned."

- Provide accurate information and demonstrate desired action. Present information in a culturally appropriate manner.

- Recognize the dynamic state of knowledge and information in the field, stay abreast of, and appropriately use new information.

- Emphasize prevention, for example, in explaining to homeowners and grounds managers how to minimize use of pesticides and fertilizers.

- Seek continual learning, educational, and mentoring opportunities.

C2. <u>Communicate</u>: The capacity to effectively communicate risk and exchange information with colleagues, other practitioners, clients, policy-makers, interest groups, media, and the public through public speaking, print and electronic media, and interpersonal relations.

Examples:

- Handle all forms of communication promptly, politely, and professionally. These include letter and e-mail correspondence, telephone calls, site visits, group discussions, meetings, and presentations.

- Explain complicated issues and procedures simply and accurately. Identify the target audience and deliver the message appropriately.

- Handle interactions with the public and media using tactful, objective, non confrontational, culturally sensitive language. Interactions include receiving complaints and providing feedback to complainants, sharing information with clients and citizen groups, motivating clients to bring about desired changes, and resolving conflicts within a community on the use of natural resources, and presenting to a hearing officer in court a case against a restaurant that has been closed.

- Seek opportunities for public speaking to broaden the audience on environmental health issues. Examples include making speeches to school groups on food safety or to swimming pool and apartment building owners and managers, conducting food handler training and giving presentations to the Chamber of Commerce. Public speaking skills can be enhanced through a variety of resources, including participation in Toastmasters, learning PowerPoint and other slide presentation software, and mentoring.

C3. <u>Conflict Resolution</u>: The capacity to facilitate resolution of conflicts within the agency, in the community, and with regulated parties.

Examples:

- Know when conflict resolution can be used and when it cannot, either because of a lack of authority or because of the intractable nature of the conflict. Recognize the limits of authority and flexibility. Typical conflicts involve complaint investigations or disagreements over a regulation, where clients might inform the practitioner that they have conducted business a certain way for years and see no reason to change, then announce their intention to seek redress from elected officials.
- Use effective listening skills.
- Exhibit respect for diversity.
- Understand the history and context of the conflict.
- Identify the nucleus of problem, separate from symptoms.
- Find common ground and areas of agreement (as well as non-negotiable areas).
- Determine the willingness of the parties involved to negotiate and promote that willingness.
- Obtain the necessary resources to resolve conflict (e.g., use of facilitators or mediators).

C4. <u>Marketing</u>: The capacity to articulate basic concepts of environmental health and public health and convey an understanding of their value and importance to clients and the public.

Examples:

- Articulate the goals, purposes, problems, and needs of environmental health.

- Provide solutions to environmental health problems that obtain support from clients and increase their understanding of environmental health issues and concerns.

- Explain the rationale for environmental health regulatory requirements and the value produced by a healthy environment (e.g., less disease, lower health care costs).

PART III: TRAITS AND CHARACTERISTICS OF AN EFFECTIVE ENVIRONMENTAL HEALTH PRACTITIONER

The group identified additional traits and characteristics thought to be common among effective environmental health practitioners. The group after identifying these traits and characteristics wanted to document them for use by managers, academicians and practitioners as important to the practice of local environmental health.

- Positive attitude
- Versatility and flexibility
- Practical perspective and common sense
- Strong principles and ethics
- Practitioner integrity
- Strong work ethic
- Tenacity
- Willingness to learn
- Focus on fair solutions
- Collaborative spirit
- Willingness to embrace change
- Involvement with community
- Calmness during conflict
- Understanding of other points of view
- Ability to observe
- Focus on team accomplishments
- Appropriate appearance and body language
- Ability to lead
- Big-picture perspective
- Respect for diversity
- Knowledge of when to ask for help

PART IV: NEXT STEPS

Panelists developed a list of next steps and opportunities for publicizing and using the environmental health competencies presented in this document. Panelists emphasized the importance of obtaining feedback, revising the competencies, and ensuring their use. Panelists suggested the following means of accomplishing these goals:

- Widely distribute this document in print and on the Internet, with links to represented organizations.

- Obtain endorsement of competencies by affiliated associations. Ensure that associations distribute the document and/or competencies to their members.

- Publish the competencies and accompanying articles in practitioner journals (e.g., CDC's *MMWR, Journal of Environmental Health*).

- Present findings and recommendations to credentialing boards of ASPH, NEHA, NALBOH, NACCHO/ASTHO, CSTE, APHL, and IAFP.

- Develop platforms to speak about competencies at conferences, meetings, and other educational and networking opportunities.

- Identify a mechanism to find and disseminate training programs and products.

- Determine which of the competencies can be added to curricula and disseminated and which should be developed as continuing education modules.

- Review past efforts and understand why other credentialing and competency efforts have succeeded or failed. Analyze past efforts to disseminate information and build on successful elements.

- Return technical and core competencies to NEHA and the credentialing process.

- Identify funding to allow work to continue toward implementation.

- Find a mechanism to develop an "association of associations"--a coalition comprising the organizations represented by the panelists and others. APHA's legislative group in this area, the National Environmental Health Coalition, may be a possible umbrella group.

- Link this competencies document with the NEHA credentialing process in one document.

Revised June 27, 2001

PART V: APPENDICES A-G

Revised June 27, 2001

Appendix A

Environmental Health Competency Project
Expert Panel Members

Ned E. Baker, MPH (panelist)
National Association of Local Boards
of Health
1021 Melrose Street
Bowling Green, OH 43402
419-352-0370 (B)
419-353-6278 (F)
email: njbaker@wcnet.org

Daniel Boatright, PhD (panelist)
Association of Schools of Public Health
University of Oklahoma
Health Science Center
School of Public Health
801 NE 13th
Oklahoma City, OH 73104
405-271-2070 (B)
405-271-1971 (F)
email: daniel-boatright@ouhsc.edu

Gary Coleman (panelist)
President
National Environmental Health
Association
720 S. Colorado Blvd.,
South Tower, Suite 970
Denver. CO 80246-1925
303-756-9090 (B)
303-691-9490 (F)
email: gary.e.coleman@us.ul.com

Trenton Davis, DrPH (panelist)
Association of Environmental Health
Academic Programs
East Carolina University
Department of Environmental Health
School of Allied Health Sciences
Greenville, NC 27858-4353
252-328-4456 (B)
252-328-0380 (F)
email: davist@mail.ecu.edu

Thomas S. Dunlop, BA, REHS (panelist)
National Association of County & City
Health Officials
Director
Aspen/Pitkin Environmental Health
Dept.
130 S. Galena Street
Aspen, CO 81611
970-920-5073 (B)
970-929-5074 (F)
email: tomd@ci.aspen.co.us

Steve Gradus, PhD (panelist)
Association of Public Health
Laboratories
Laboratory Director
City of Milwaukee Health Dept.
841 N. Broadway, Room 205
Milwaukee, WI 53202
414-286-3526 (B)
414-286-5098 (F)
email: sgradu@ci.mil.wi.us

Rebecca A. Head, PhD, DABT (panelist)
American Public Health Association
Director
Washtenaw County Environmental
Health &
Infrastructure Services
P. O. Box 8645
Ann Arbor, MI 48107-8645
734-
734-994-2459 (F)
email: headr@co.washtenaw.mi.us

23

Mel Knight, REHS, BS (panelist)
National Conference of Local
Environmental
 Health Administrators
Sacramento County Environmental
Health
 Management Department
8475 Jackson Road, Suite 200
Sacramento, CA 95826
916-875-1732 (B)
916-875-8588 (F)
email:
knightm@emd.co.sacramento.ca.us

Bela Matyas, MD, MPH (panelist)
(for Henry Anderson, MD)
Council of State & Territorial
Epidemiologists
Division of Epidemiology and
Immunization
Massachusetts Department of Public
Health
State Lab Institute
305 South Street, Room 506
Jamaica Plain, MA 02130-3597
617-983-6847 (B)
email: bela.matyas@state.ma.us

Carol Miller, MPH (panelist)
National Rural Health Association
Frontier Education Center
HCR 65, Box 126
Ojo Sarco, NM 87521
505-689-2361 (B)
505-689-2329 (F)
email: frontierus@frontierus.org

**Robert W. Powitz, PhD, AAS, BSA,
MPH (panelist)**
American Academy of Sanitarians
8 Pheasant Hill Lane., P.O. Box 501
Old Saybrook, CT 06475
860-388-0893 (B)
860-388-9566 (F)
email: sanitarian@juno.com

Leonard F. Rice, RS, MES (panelist)
Association of State & Territorial Health
Officials
South Carolina Dept. of Health and
Environmental Control
Edisto Health District
P.O. Box 1126
Orangeburg, SC 29116
803-536-9060 (B)
802-536-9118
email: ricelf@orngbg60.dhe.state.sc.us

Gloria Swick, MSA (panelist)
International Association for Food
Protection
Health Commissioner
Perry County Health Department
P.O. Box 230
New Lexington, OH 43764
740-342-5179 (B)
740-342-1276 (F)
email: pchd@netpluscom.com

Presenters and Staff

Thomas A. Burke, PhD, MPH
Johns Hopkins University
624 N. Broadway, Room 484
Baltimore, MD 21205
410-955-1604 (B)
410-614-2797 (F)
email: tburke@jhsph.edu

Larry Gordon
Adjunct Professor
Political Science Department
Social Science Bldg., 2nd Floor
University of New Mexico
Albuquerque, MN 87131-1121
505-277-7761 (B)
505-277-2821 (F)
email: eljaygee@unm.edu

Revised June 27, 2001

Petrona Lee, MS, RS
Manager
Environmental Health Services
City of Bloomington
2215 West Old Shakopee Road
Bloomington, MN 55431-3096
612-948-8970 (B)
612-948-8949 (F)
email: plee@ci.bloomington.mn.us

Heidi M. Klein, MSEH (Facilitator)
32 Wildwood Drive
Essex, VT 05452
802-879-9661 (B)
802-879-9661 (F)
email: heidimklein@hotmail.com

**Patrick O. Bohan, RS, MS, MSEH
(Project Officer)**
National Center for Environmental Health
4770 Buford Highway, NE
Mailstop F28
Atlanta, GA 30341
770-488-7303 (B)
770-488-7310 (F)
email: pfb3@cdc.gov

Annette Ferebee, MPH (APHA Staff)
Project Director
American Public Health Association
800 I Street, NW
Washington, DC 20001-3710
202-777-2494 (B)
202-777-2533 (F)
email: annette.ferebee@apha.org

**Julie Desai, MPH Candidate (APHA
Intern)**
Environmental Health Intern
American Public Health Association
800 I Street, NW
Washington, DC 20001-3710
202-777-2494 (B)
202-777-2533 (F)
email: annette.ferebee@apha.org

Gilah Langner (writer)
Stetton Associates, Inc.
3035 Porter Street, NW
Washington, DC 20008
202-364-3006 (B)
202-364-3806 (F)
email: langner@stretton.com

Revised June 27, 2001

Appendix B

SUMMARY OF EXPERT PANEL DISCUSSION

Dr. Thomas A. Burke (Johns Hopkins University) opened the Expert Panel meeting on the evening of February 28, 2000, with a review of his work and that of the Pew Trust. He presented incentives for attracting students to schools of public health, opportunities for fostering collaboration across disciplines, and ways of encouraging mentoring. Dr. Burke noted the need to "come together as a discipline" to obtain the funding and support that environmental health deserves

> *Professor Gordon called on environmental health leaders to take an active role not just in defining competencies but also in strengthening the organizations, funding, and standards that produce environmental health practitioners*

Professor Larry Gordon (University of New Mexico) summarized the training and practice of environmental health and protection practitioners. Environmental health, noted Professor Gordon, is the single largest component of the field of public health, accounting for roughly half of expenditures and numbers of personnel. Few public health leaders are aware of this, however, because the vast majority of environmental health activities are located outside public health departments and are not calculated into public health expenditures. Public health and environmental health have been on a slowly diverging path, with the practice of public health gravitating toward personal health care, and environmental health aligning itself with environmental quality and conservation. Accredited schools and programs do not adequately address the need and potential market for undergraduate and graduate environmental health practitioners. Professor Gordon's recommendations included promoting competencies in emerging areas of environmental health, strengthening accreditation requirements, and encouraging mentoring by persons in leadership positions.

26

Petrona Lee (Bloomington, Minnesota's Environmental Health Services), focused on core competency training for the environmental health practitioner. She decried the splintering of environmental health functions across a variety of local departments--for example, assigning firefighters to inspect houses between calls. Where environmental health practitioners work under supervisors who have no environmental health background, in-service training is less likely to be standardized. She encouraged pay-scale parity for environmental health practitioners and increasing opportunities for continuing education and enriching interchange with the scientific community.

Dr. Mohammad Akhter, (American Public Health Association [APHA]), opened the morning session of the Expert Panel on February 29, noting that environmental health is a priority for APHA's 55,000 members who work in dozens of different disciplines. Public health cannot be improved unless people in all disciplines work together. For many years, APHA and other organizations have provided continuing education to public health practitioners, focused primarily on technical aspects. Whether these competencies are sufficient for people in environmental health positions is questionable. Dr. Akhter noted that the aim of this Expert Panel meeting is to develop a consensus that will help change the education and continuing education curricula and may lead to certification.

Susan West (APHA Environment Section), urged the panel to cut across its technical expertise and disciplines to move this initiative forward. Encouraging the group to review and comment on the APHA Environment Section's Strategic Plan (http://www.apha.org/private/splan99), she noted that several of the goal areas in the strategic plan relate to environmental health practice. She hoped that the Environmental Health Competency Project, by convening organizations and agencies with similar goals and interests yet with little history of collaboration, would be a concrete step in establishing a leadership role for APHA in the arena of environmental health practice.

Facilitator Heidi Klein focused the meeting on the competencies that make a person an effective environmental health practitioner within a public health context. She noted that the NEHA has defined technical competencies for an environmental health specialist.

Revised June 27, 2001

The panel's effort is intended to complement NEHA's work by focusing on core competencies and to identify the key competencies needed to apply those skills in local public health practice.

A. Specifying the Target

The competencies were selected to apply to environmental health practitioners to functions effectively on the job.

Panelists agreed that their goal was to outline the **core competencies that an environmental health practitioner will need to be effective as part of line staff in a local public health agency.**

The Expert Panel emphasized that these competencies are not the minimum requirements for hiring an entry-level environmental health practitioner. The competencies are those expected of an environmental health practitioner after he or she had worked the job and had received on-the-job training and perhaps continuing education.

Environmental health practitioners may need to develop additional competencies as they advance in their careers. As environmental health practitioners reach managerial levels, they are likely to need specific management skills that are not covered here. However, not everyone aspires to be an administrator, and management skills are not generally needed for line staff positions unless an individual is working in an agency where he or she operates solo. In some areas of the country, notably New England states, an environmental health practitioner may be the only employee of the health agency. In Massachusetts, for example, about 10% of the counties have only one person (sometimes part-time) addressing environmental and public health issues. By default, this person functions simultaneously as an environmental health practitioner, health administrator, and manager.

Revised June 27, 2001

> *Panelists reiterated that they are not trying to specify what an environmental health practitioner has to do, but instead are outlining the competencies that will make an environmental health practitioner more effective on the job.*

Panelists discussed the variety of environmental health positions and responsibilities, even within public health agencies, ranging from food and building inspections to sewage disposal and site remediation. Some competencies presuppose a course in the subject; others are more a matter of exposure and awareness of the subject matter. Although it may not be in environmental health, the environmental health practitioner should have at least an undergraduate degree. Some states are beginning to express a preference for environmental health training for positions involving environmental health. Some states require only a high school diploma for sanitarians; in Ohio, on the other hand, a sanitarian-in-training needs to have at least 45 hours of science and a four year degree, followed by a highly structured schedule for passing competency tests over a five year period.

Because some competencies are developed over time, specifying them can be difficult. Panelists pointed out that certain competencies come with maturity, experience, and training and that they cannot be expected in an entry-level position. Problem solving is an example. Although inspectors must be able to make decisions and solve problems, they may also need to make mistakes before they learn how to handle certain situations. Panelists reiterated that they are not trying to specify what an environmental health practitioner has to do but are outlining the competencies that will make an environmental health practitioner more effective. Identifying these competencies will be useful to a variety of people and organizations, including school administrators, organizations offering continuing education courses and managers in public health agencies who train entry-level persons.

Finally, panelists were sensitive to the issue of whether their recommendations can realistically be met. Many state governments no longer support continuing education or in-service training and often do not support out-of-state travel. Although opportunities exist for distance learning and other ways of providing information to people, not disadvantaging environmental health practitioners who have no access to training is important. Panelists expressed concern that once competencies are defined, they may someday be used to grade employees, placing rural staff especially at a disadvantage. The panelists hoped that these competencies would serve as goals and guides to positively influence training and work expectation. Panelists stopped short of recommending these competencies be used in evaluating performance.

Before examining specific competencies, the Expert Panel reviewed the results of an informal e-mail survey of NACCHO members about key environmental health competencies. Responses were received from 55 of 200 potential respondents, representing different classifications of health departments. Respondents generally agreed that core competencies should include: environmental epidemiology, environmental science, general communication skills, public health, risk communication skills, risk assessment skills, and sanitation. Other topics for which there was substantial agreement included bio-statistics, managerial and organizational skills, communicable disease/chronic disease control, community health, public relations, and risk management skills. Overall, more agreement existed among rural observers than among metro respondents, probably because of the diversity of urban environments and the greater tendency to compartmentalize environmental health into different areas.

> *The panelists hoped these competencies would serve as goals and guides to positively influence training and work expectation*

B. Refining the List of Competencies

Panelists narrowed the lists of potential core competencies to a recommended set. They discussed both the content of each of the competencies and the meaning of the title. They recognized that certain words mean different things to different people. For example, some panelists questioned whether the competency "Policy Development" implied that an environmental health practitioner should be able to go to the Board of Health and argue for a particular policy. This task probably would not be relevant at an entry-level position. Alternatively, does it mean the need to understand what policies are in effect, how they are formed and implemented, and how they can be changed? Although these tasks are all essential for working effectively, they also represent a basic "knowledge" part of the job rather than a competency. On the other hand, front-line staff, especially solo practitioners, may be involved in policy development. For example, they might consult with one another on whether certain regulations (e.g., tattoo regulations) are in place in their communities and how the regulations were developed. Panelists ultimately determined that the term "Policy Development" itself is vague and that pieces of it are incorporated in other competencies.

Some of the competencies that had been suggested before the meeting by one or more panelists were considered technical competencies and were referred to NEHA for further discussion. These included:

- Environmental and public health microbiology (separate from communicable diseases).
- Safety science. (Although NEHA covers occupational safety and health, environmental health practitioners are often called on to help with safety issues and injury prevention, especially relating to children and the elderly.)
- Bio-statistics.
- Public health laboratory science.
- Emergency response.

31

Revised June 27, 2001

Other competency suggestions that were discussed but not included in the recommended list of competencies are shown below, along with the reasons for excluding them:

Competency	Reason
Managerial and administrative skills	Not required of line staff
Strategic planning	Not required of line staff
Personnel management	Not required of line staff
Effective delegation	Not required of line staff
Financial planning	Covered under Work Planning
Environmental engineering	Technical skill; "plan review" aspects are covered under NEHA
Sustainable technologies	Technical aspects are covered under NEHA
Energy production, resource utilization, transportation methodology, product design and development	Part of concept of environmental health planning, referred to NEHA
Geographic information systems	Technical area
Epidemiology concepts	Technical area, covered under NEHA
Decision theory	Technical area
Software	Included under Computer/Information Technology competency. Specific software packages are specified by each agency.
Environmental economics	Technical area

Appendix C

Typical Responsibilities of Environmental Health and Protection Programs

Environmental health and protection practitioners should educate, think and act in terms of risk assessment, risk communication, and risk management activities to protect human health and the environment relating to the following problems:

Ambient air quality
    Indoor air quality, including radon
    Water pollution control, including thermal pollution
    Safe drinking water, including public, semi-public and private sources
    Noise pollution
    Radiation, including ionizing and non ionizing
Food, including eating and drinking establishments
    Food processing establishments
    Fish and shellfish
    Pure food
    Meat
    Poultry
    Milk
Industrial hygiene
Childhood lead poisoning
Acid deposition
Disaster planning and response
Cross-connection elimination
Healthy housing
Institutional environmental control, including schools, health-care facilities, correction facilities, and day care centers
Recreational area environmental control, including swimming pools, campgrounds, and beaches.
Solid waste management
Hazardous waste management, including hazardous spills
Vector control, including insects and rodents
Pesticide control
Toxic chemical control, including community right-to-know
On-site liquid waste disposal
Unintentional injury control
Bioterrorism
Global environmental issues such as global warming, stratospheric ozone depletion and planetary toxification

Program activities to solve or ameliorate the foregoing problems include: surveillance regulation, including: warnings, hearings, permits, grading, compliance schedules, variances, injunctions, administrative and judicial penalties, embargoes, environmental impact requirements, sampling, education, inspection, complaint response, consultation, networking and community involvement, pollution prevention, design and plan review, economic and social incentives, public information, and prioritization

Environmental health planning for prevention through effective involvement during the planning, design and decision stages of energy production and utilization, land use, transportation systems, resource development and consumption, and product and facility design

Environmental health and protection support services include: epidemiology, laboratory services, legal services, *GIS*, personnel training, information technology, public policy design and implementation, marketing, research, strategic planning,

Environmental health and protection practitioners should have a vision, a philosophy and a comprehensive
    understanding of environmental health and protection, rather than the inspection and reaction approach.

Appendix D

Technical Competencies Covered in NEHA's Registered Environmental Health Specialist/ Registered Sanitarian Exam

- Basic Environmental Health and Protection
- Basic Sciences:
  -- Toxicology
  -- Physics
  -- Chemistry
  -- Geology
  -- Biology
- Epidemiology:
  -- Environmental
  -- Occupational
- Communicable/Chronic Disease
- Environmental Law (statutes and regulations)
- Risk Assessment
- Risk Management

Appendix E

Content Areas of NEHA's Registered Environmental Health Specialist/Registered Sanitarian (REHS/RS)Exam

The REHS/RS exam is based on the following content areas. Beside each subject heading is the approximate percentage of questions in that content area on the exam.

1. **Statutes and Regulations   6%**
   Knowledge of legal authority, law about inspections, agency administrative actions (e.g., embargo, seizure, nuisance abatement), federal environmental health acts, laws, agencies, and regulations.

2. **Food Protection   15%**
   Knowledge of inspection/investigation procedures of food establishments. Knowledge of food safety principles, protection, quality, and storage. Knowledge of temporary food service events. Knowledge of proper food transport.

3. **Potable Water   9%**
   Knowledge of sanitary survey principles regarding potential or existing water systems and watersheds. Understanding of testing/sampling methods, water supply systems, water treatment processes, and diseases associated with contaminated water.

4. **Wastewater   10%**
   Knowledge of inspection/investigation procedures of wastewater systems. Knowledge of soil characteristics and analysis methods, land use issues, wastewater treatment systems and processes, and disease-causing organisms associated with wastewater.

5. **Solid and Hazardous Waste   10%**
   Knowledge of waste-management systems, waste classifications, landfill methods, hazardous waste disposal methods, and health risks associated with poor waste management.

6. **Hazardous Materials   5%**
   Knowledge of inspections and investigations of hazardous materials, self-protection procedures, and types of hazardous materials.

7. **Vectors, Pests, and Weeds   8%**
   Knowledge of control methods for vectors, pests, and weeds; life cycle; different types of vectors, pests, and weeds; diseases and organisms associated with vectors, pests, and weeds; and public education methods.

8. **Radiation Protection   4%**
   Knowledge of inspections/investigations of radiation hazards, types of radiation, common sources of exposure, protection methods, health risks of radiation

exposure, and testing equipment and sampling methods used to detect radiation.

9. **Occupational Safety and Health   4%**
Knowledge of inspection/investigation procedures of occupational settings, common health and safety hazards at worksites, and general OSHA principles.

10. **Air Quality and Noise   4%**
Knowledge of inspection and investigation procedures to assess ambient air quality and environmental noise, air pollution sources, air and noise sampling methods and equipment, air and noise pollution control equipment and techniques, and health risks associated with poor air quality and excessive noise.

11. **Housing   6%**
Knowledge of inspection and investigation procedures of public and private housing and mobile home and recreational vehicle parks, health and safety risks of substandard housing, housing codes, heating, ventilation, and cooling systems, child safety hazards such as lead, and utility connections.

12. **Institutions and Licensed Establishments   9%**
Knowledge of the health hazards and sanitation problems commonly associated with correctional facilities, medical facilities, licensed establishments (tanning salons, massage clinics, tattoo parlors, and cosmetology salons) child-care facilities and schools; common disease-causing organisms and transmission modes; epidemiology; and heating, ventilation, and cooling systems.

13. **Swimming Pools and Recreational Facilities   7%**
Knowledge of inspection and investigation procedures for swimming pools and spas, recreational areas and facilities, amusement parks, temporary mass gatherings (e.g., concerts, county fairs, etc.). Knowledge of common organisms and resultant diseases associated with swimming pools and spas, water treatment systems, water chemistry, safety issues, and sampling and test methods.

14. **Disaster Sanitation   3%**
Knowledge of disaster preparation, site management of disaster situations, and post-disaster management. Knowledge of emergency response procedures, chain of command, supply needs, temporary shelter and facilities and services, and remediation methods.

Appendix F

SETTING THE CONTEXT:
ENVIRONMENTAL HEALTH PRACTITIONER COMPETENCIES
Presented to
American Public Health Association - National Center for Environmental Health
Workshop
Washington, DC
February 28, 2000
by
Larry Gordon, University of New Mexico

Important change requires time and persistence. Inasmuch as I have articulated many of the observations and recommendations that I am making today for a number of years, I offer the following quotation attributed to Albert Schweitzer:

> *No ray of sunshine is ever lost, but the green which it awakes into existence needs time to sprout, and is not always granted to the sower to see the harvest. All that is worth anything is done in faith.*

CURRENT STATE OF AFFAIRS

- Environmental health and protection is a high priority issue in our society. It is demanded by the public, the media and political leaders, and is widely considered to be an entitlement.

- Environmental health and protection is a profoundly complex, multifaceted, multidisciplinary, and interdisciplinary field of endeavor engaged in by a wide spectrum of disciplines, professions and others within a complex array of public and private organizations.

- The field of public health practice has evolved into at least **two major systems** for the delivery of comprehensive public health services at the state and federal levels, the major areas being personal public health and environmental health and protection.

- Environmental health and protection is the responsibility of numerous agencies at the federal, state and local levels, as well as in the private sector.

- At the state level, 90 to 95% of environmental health and protection activities are assigned to agencies other than health departments, and there appears to be a similar trend at the local level.

- Expenditures and numbers of personnel for environmental health and protection account for roughly 50% of the field of public health practice and is, therefore, the

largest single component of the field of public health. Few public health leaders acknowledge this because the annual reports of the Public Health Foundation do not include the expenditures of the 90 to 95% of environmental health and protection activities that are not in health departments. This under-representation of environmental health and protection expenditures continues to make environmental health and protection appear to be but a bit player in the field of public health.

Definitions are essential. In the absence of standard definitions, every group confuses and garbles the issues by re-inventing the wheel. **A product cannot be uniformly understood or marketed if we don't know whether we're dealing with a buggy whip or a rocket ship**. Therefore, I will define and comment on a few key terms.

The standard definition for **environmental health and protection** was developed for the widely peer reviewed "Report on the Future of Environmental Health", and was used in the primary reference document for this meeting. This definition should provide a framework for our discussions.

> *Environmental health and protection is the art and science of protecting against environmental factors that may adversely impact human health or the ecological balances essential to long-term human health and environmental quality. Such factors include, but are not limited to: air, food and water contaminants; radiation; toxic chemicals; wastes; disease vectors; safety hazards; and habitat alterations.*

Most environmental health and protection practitioners may be classified as **environmental health and protection professionals**, or as **professionals in environmental health and protection**. All are essential components of any comprehensive effort.

> *Environmental health and protection professionals are those who have been adequately educated in the various environmental health and protection technical (programmatic) components, as well as in epidemiology, biostatistics, toxicology, management, public policy, risk assessment and reduction, risk communication, environmental law, social dynamics and environmental economics.*

> *Professionals in environmental health and protection include other essential personnel such as chemists, geologists, biologists, meteorologists, physicists, physicians, economists, engineers, attorneys, planners, epidemiologists, social scientists, public administrators and planners.*

Probably less than 5% of the workforce are environmental health professionals. Few **environmental health professionals** are utilized by agencies other than health departments. But even in health departments, most environmental health and protection personnel are **professionals in environmental health** rather than environmental health professionals.

It is not necessary that all environmental health and protection personnel be educated as **environmental health professionals**. Many essential roles are best filled by **professionals in environmental health** such as those previously iterated. However, personnel other than environmental health professionals would benefit from continuing education in key environmental health competencies such as epidemiology, toxicology, risk assessment, risk communication, risk management, as well as an inculcation of an environmental health vision and philosophy. The philosophy must include an understanding of the scope, values, goals and potential of environmental health and protection. Whatever disciplines and professions are involved, they must be competent to do a public health job.

Many environmental health and protection professionals appear reluctant to incur the controversies and risks inherent in top policy and leadership roles. Leadership positions do not offer career protection beyond the ability of an individual to earn the respect and support of peers, subordinates, the public, the media and elected officials. Leadership belongs to no group by divine right or genetic proclivity.

While there are differences in the programmatic responsibilities assigned local, state and federal environmental health and protection agencies, the basic competencies necessary to engage effectively in the various programs are the same, varying only in degree of emphasis. Practitioners should be competent to practice in the **field** of environmental health and protection rather than any specific type or level of agencies in the public **or** private sectors so that they may achieve career flexibility, effectiveness and success. Many practitioners have worked at the local **and** state levels, some at the local, state **and** federal levels, and others in the private sector as well. State level practitioners benefit by having had **prior** local experience, federal practitioners benefit by having had prior state and/or local experience, and all would benefit from experience in the private sector.

Public health is not in disarray as the Institute of Medicine suggested. It is far more diverse and complex than the public health agency model the IOM would create. Environmental health and protection goals are increasingly being addressed by agencies other than the evolving type of health departments. The practice of public health other than environmental health and protection is gravitating closer to a partnership with health care, while environmental health and protection is aligning more closely with environmental quality and conservation agencies.

Accredited schools and programs are not adequately addressing the need and potential market for undergraduate or graduate practitioners. Environmental health and protection policies and priorities are the responsibility of those engaged at the more rarefied administrative and policy levels of the public and private sector. Until such personnel are made available by our nation's schools of public health and environmental health science and protection programs, most leadership and policy positions will continue to be filled by individuals possessing other credentials. This leadership and policy niche is no longer being addressed by schools of public health. Schools of public health, once the incubators for public health practitioners, have been gravitating away from developing environmental health and protection practitioners as they follow the money trail toward emphasizing basic science research and health care rather than public health practice. Courses in health law are usually health care law, courses in health administration are usually health care administration, courses in health policy are usually health care policy, and courses in health financing and economics are usually health care financing and economics. Competencies necessary for the field of environmental health and protection **practice** have not been an important consideration, and course content in environmental health and protection finance, policy, law, administration, and a philosophy and vision of environmental health is somewhere between rare and non-existent.

Most environmental health faculty in schools of public health are narrowly oriented basic science researchers rather than academically qualified generalists or practitioners. This change is reflected by the type of graduates, their competencies, and the nature of their careers. Academicians become mentors and role models, and most schools of public health are not providing role models and mentors for those who might otherwise enter the field of practice rather than narrow basic science fields, teaching and research.

Additionally, the Council on Education for Public Health has not addressed relevant competencies for environmental health practitioners even though specific recommendations have been offered repeatedly.

Accreditation criteria of the National Environmental Health Science and Protection Accreditation Council are more relevant to the field of practice than are those of the Council on Education for Public Health. Undergraduates produced by NEHSPAC accredited programs generally possess the competencies needed for practice at the entrance and journeyman levels. Unfortunately, there are only three NEHSPAC accredited graduate programs.

Do you ever wonder why institutions such as the Kennedy School rather than schools of public health and accredited environmental health science and protection programs are preparing students for environmental health and protection policy and leadership roles?

SOME PERSONAL COMMENTS

I have enjoyed a rewarding career in public and environmental health, commencing as an entrance grade sanitarian and retiring as a state Cabinet Secretary for Health and Environment. But more significant than having titles; creating agencies, laws, ordinances; holding offices and receiving recognition, I am most proud of my successes in mentoring scores of professionals who went on to significant roles and achievements. By placing a high value on competency, I encouraged dozens of personnel to earn graduate degrees in public or environmental health. At one time, I was in the enviable position of having individuals with such graduate credentials as Director of the State Environmental Agency, Director of the State Public Health Agency, and Director of the State Scientific Laboratory System. Importantly, all had started at the local level. In the state environmental agency, the Director as well as every division director and district manager had an MPH or closely related degree. I also developed and gained passage of a state law requiring that directors of local health departments have a MPH. For me, those were days of Camelot.

That was at a time when schools of public health produced professionals for the **field** of practice. I owe much of any success I may have had to the basic competencies, vision and philosophy I acquired at a school of public health many years ago. Most of my personnel went on to greener pastures. Last month, two of these long ago protégés called me for lunch. I want to tell you a little about these two as examples of the potential of individuals having the necessary competencies for the **field** of practice.

I hired both right out of college as entrance grade sanitarians when I was Director of the Albuquerque Health Department. Both worked in food protection. I admonished that everyone should be re-potted every few years so as not to become root bound. I encouraged both to earn their MPHs. I recruited both back to New Mexico while I was Director of the New Mexico Environmental Improvement Agency. One became Director of Field Operations, one became Director of OSHA. At later dates, both became Director of the Environmental Improvement Agency. A new Governor eventually left both with the need to seek greener pastures --- the potential price of leadership ventures.

One subsequently became Santa Fe City Manager, Vice President of the University of Arizona, Deputy Assistant Secretary of Defense for Environment, a key position with BDM International, Director of Environmental Management for Los Alamos National Laboratories, and was recently recruited to become Vice President for Material Stewardship for Kaiser-Hill -- the contractor responsible for cleaning up Rocky Flats because he has the competency and confidence to get the job done. Tom Baca can't resist a challenge.

The other was subsequently appointed Regional EPA Director of Environmental Services, resigned to become Director of Environmental Quality for the State of Arizona, a new Governor intervened, and Russell Rhodes is now Director of Environmental Affairs for Public Service Company of New Mexico.

Both practitioners continue to achieve and enjoy their careers utilizing competencies gained while earning an MPH during the days when schools of public health were professional schools rather than research institutions and had a priority of educating practitioners and emphasizing environmental health.

I could cite numerous similar examples, but I have mentioned Tom Baca and Russell Rhoades to emphasize the benefits of being competent to practice in the **field** of environmental health and protection, and to stress the importance of mentoring as a leadership responsibility.

SOME COMPETENCY ASSURANCE RECOMMENDATIONS

Revised June 27, 2001

- Enactment of a federal **"Environmental Health Science and Protection Education and Training Act"** such as that included in the HRSA report *Educating Environmental Health Science and Protection Professionals.*

- An effective **education and training coordinating mechanism** involving appropriate federal agencies.

- Ensure that environmental health **data collected by the Public Health Foundation include expenditures of environmental health and protection** agencies in addition to health departments so as to accurately reflect the size and importance of the field of practice.

- Admonish that practitioners be competent to practice in the **field of environmental health and protection** to ensure career mobility, effectiveness and success.

- **Ensure competencies in ecological and global environmental** issues because these problems will determine the future of public health.

- Ensure competencies in the complex and essential mix of **regulatory methodologies** in addition to the better accepted competencies in epidemiology, risk assessment, risk communication, risk management, and toxicology.

- Ensure that accredited schools **and programs** produce qualified **graduate** level personnel who are competent, willing and available to vie for top level **managerial and policy positions** in the complex spectrum of possible roles if we are to again establish leadership in the field of environmental health and protection. Students aspiring to **leadership roles** must be inculcated with such skills as management, public policy, planning, political science, public finance, organizational behavior, interpersonal and public relations, and marketing, as well as a vision and philosophy of environmental health and protection.

- Ensure that **schools and programs** utilize **academically qualified environmental health practitioners** who will serve as role models and mentors among their mix of faculty.

- Schools of public health could begin regaining environmental health leadership by changing school titles and emphases to **schools of public and environmental health.** The advantages would be manifold in terms of attracting money, students and political support.

- Create a **Division of Environmental Health within HRSA** as a step toward emphasizing the size and importance of environmental health and providing necessary training funds.

- The Council on Education for Public Health should **strengthen environmental health and protection accreditation** requirements.

42

- Ensure that **continuing education** needs of our nation's environmental health and protection workforce is a priority at all levels of the public and private sectors, as well as in academia. Formal education is inadequate by itself, and does not provide personnel all the evolving knowledge and skills required.

And finally,

- Encourage **mentoring** by those in leadership positions to build on the competencies inculcated in formal education. **Personnel must be encouraged, supported, and counseled to achieve, and to be all they can be.**

Environmental health leaders must take the **lead** not only in specifying the competencies of the environmental health and protection workforce, **but more importantly**, taking steps to **ensure the necessary measures to make it all happen such as suggested above!** Otherwise, we will **continue** talking to each other, **continue** believing that talking to each other is accomplishing something, and **continue to be shackled by inaction** Do not assume that others will look after the competency needs of the workforce. Achieving competency goals will depend on environmental health and protection leaders fulfilling their responsibilities.

Appendix G

Resources

APHA. Environment Section Strategic Plan. Adopted by section leadership-
March 9, 1999.

American Industrial Hygiene Association and Hughes, C. Industrial Hygiene: Work
Force Characteristics:

Employment, Education & Practice. July 1992. USDHHS. HRSA.

Association of Schools of Public Health and Gordon, L. J. Education Environmental
Health Science &

Protection Professionals: Problems, Challenges & Recommendations. USDHHS.
HRSA. 1991.

Baker, E. L., Brown, C. K., and Gerzoff, R. B. Full-Time Employees of U.S. Local
Health Departments,

1992-1993. J Public Health Management Practice, 1999 5(3), 1-9.

Baker, E. L., and Gerzoff, R. B. The Use of Scaling Techniques to Analyze U. S. Local
Health Department

Staffing Structures, 1992-1993. 1998 Proceedings of the Section on Government
Statistics and

Section on Social Statistics of the American Statistical Association.

Blacconiere, M. J and Oleckno, W. A. Job Satisfaction Among Environmental Health
Professionals: An

Examination of Descriptors, Correlates and Predictors. January/February 1993. J. E. H.
Volume 55, Number 4.

Boatright, D. T. Environmental Health Partnerships: A Formula for Success. June 1998.
Central Regional Workshop. USDHHS. HRSA.

Boatright, D. T. Environmental Health Partnerships: A Formula for Success. June 1998.
Western Regional Workshop. USDHHS. HRSA.

Boatright, D. T. Environmental Health Partnerships: A Formula for Success. June 1998.
Eastern Regional Workshop. USDHHS. HRSA.

Bock, S. F., and White. L. E. Environmental Health Model Internship Guidelines. September 1995. USDHHS. HRSA.

Brown, C., Fraser, M., Milne, T., Gerzoff, R., and Richards, T. Preliminary Results from the 1997 Profile of Local Health Departments. Presentation/Poster.

Brown, C., Fraser, M., Milne, T., Gerzoff, R., and Richards, T. A Snap-Shot of Local Public Health Agencies: The 1997 NACCHO Profile.

Burke, T. A., Shalauta, N. M., Tran, Nga. L., and Gordon, L. Blue Print for Education & Training; The Crossroads Colloquium: An Examination of the Educational Needs for Environmental Health and Protection. Final Report. PHS Contract Number 102HR960317P. USDHHS. HRSA.

Burke, T. A., Shalauta, N. M., Tran, Nga. L., and Stern, B. S. The Environmental Web: A National Profile of the State Infrastructure for Environmental Health and Protection. J Public Health Management Practice. 1997. 3(2), 1-12.

Burke, T. A. Tran, N. L, Shalauta, N. M. Who's in Charge? Identification of State Environmental Services: A Profile of the State Infrastructure for Environmental Health and Protection. A Final Report. March 1995. Appendix IE-State Records Appendix II-dBase Files. Contract Number 240-92-0046. USDHHS. HRSA.

Burke, T. A. Tran, N. L, Shalauta, N. M. Who's in Charge? Identification of State Environmental Services: A Profile of the State Infrastructure for Environmental Health and Protection. A Final Report. March 1995. Appendix IA-ID. Contract Number 240-92-0046. USDHHS. HRSA.

Christenson, G., Cooper, A. Suen, J. and Taylor, M. Analysis of the Current Status of Public Health Practice in Local Health Departments. PHS

Competency-Based Curriculum Group. Subcommittee on Workforce, Education, and Training. Public Health Functions Steering Committee and Working Group. Draft 12/20/96.

Conway, J. B. On the Need to Teach Science to Environmental Health Students. November/December. J. E. H. Volume 54, Number 3.29-31.

Developing an Agenda for Public Health Practice Research. Prepared for the Robert Wood Johnson Foundation. June 1999.

Evaluating Hazardous Waste Education & Training. USDHHS. HRSA and ATSDR.

The Future of Environmental Health. Part One. January/February 1993. J. E. H. Volume 55, Number 4. 28-32.

Revised June 27, 2001

The Future of Environmental Health. Part Two. March 1993. J. E. H. Volume 55, Number 5. 42-45.

Gerzoff, R. B., and Richards T. B. The Education of Local Health Department Top Executives. J Public Health Management Practice, 1997 3(4), 50-56.

Gordon, L. J. Environmental Health and Protection: Century 21 Challenges. J. E. H. January/February 1995. Volume 57, Number 6. 28-34.

Handler, A., Hall. W., Potsic, S., Nalluri, R., Turnock, B., and Vaughn, E. H. Local Health Department Effectiveness in Addressing the Core Functions of Public Health. Public Health Reports. Sept./Oct. 1994, Vol. 109, No. 5, 653-658.

Handler, A., and Turnock B. J. Local Health Department Effectiveness in Addressing the Core Functions of Public Health (CDC-ASPH Cooperative Agreements 1991-1995). One Pager.

Hatfield, T. H. The Failure of Sanitarians. March/April 1991. J. E. H. Volume 53, Number 5. Health Care Facilities Section. NEHA. Qualified Environmentalist/Sanitarian Needed in Every Health Care Facility. J. E. H. Vol. 38, No. 1. July/August 1975. 24-25.

Healthy People 2010 Objectives: Draft for Public Comment. September 15, 1998. USDHHS. OPHS. HRSA. Health Personnel in the United States. Eight Report to Congress 1991. September 1992. USDHHS. PHS. HRSA.

Hodkinson, P. and Issitt M. The Challenge of Competence: Professionalism through Vocational Education and Training. 1995. Cassell. New York.

Johnson, T. L., Stern, B. S, and Wiant, C. J. Environmental Health Survey: A Nationwide Study. January/February 1992. J. E. H. Volume 54, Number 4.

Laning, R. C. The Challenges of Environmental Health. J. E. H. Vol. 39, No. 2. Sept/Oct. 1976. 120-121.

Lustig, K. W. The Failure of Sanitarians Revisited. Guest Commentary. November/December 1992. J. E. H. Volume 55, Number 3. 63-64.

Maisch, M. and Winter, R. Professional Competence and Higher Education: The ASSET Programme. The Flamer Press. Washington, D.C.

Mansfield, B. and Mitchell, L. Towards a Competent Workforce. 1996. Gower. Vermont

Mattison, B. F. The Role of Professional Organizations in Environmental Health. Jan

46

Revised June 27, 2001

1968. Arch Environ Health. Vol 16, 116-120.

Morgan, M. T. President's Message: Environmental Health Manpower. J. E. H. Vol. 37, No. 4. . Jan/Feb 369-370.

Morgan, S. L. and Morgan, M. T. January/February 1993. Managing the Future Work Force: Trends which will Impact the Management of Environmental Health Professionals. J. E. H. Volume 55, Number 4. 20-23.

NACCHO. Environmental Health Practice. Project Fact Sheet.

NACCHO. Community Environmental Health Assessment. Project Fact Sheet.

NACCHO and CDC. 1992-1993. National Profile of Local Health Departments. 1995. National Surveillance Series.

Nolan, P. A. Public Health and Environmetnal Protection: Where will the Leadership Be? Editorial.

Oleckno, W. A. Job Satisfaction in Environmental Health: An Analysis at the Local Level. Paper Presented at the American Public Health Association, Annual Meeting, Chicago, IL. November 1999.

Pew Health Professions Commission. Critical Challenges: Revitalizing the Health Professions for the Twenty-First Century. The Third Report of the Pew Health Professions Commissions. December 1995.

Pohlit, N. The Role and Responsibilities of Professional Associations in Environmental Health. J. E. H. Vol. 37, No. 4. Jan./Feb. 1975. 387-390.

The Public Health Workforce: An Agenda for the 21st Century. Full Report of the Public Health Functions Project. USDHHS. PHS.

Public Health Practice Surveillance and Capacity Building through State & Local Health Departments. Final Report. Oct. 1994- Sept. 1995. 1-50.

Shalauta Juzych, N. Crossroads Colloquium: An Examination of the Education Needs for Environmental Health and Protection. Presentation. 1999 APHA Annual Meeting .

VanDusen, K. Women Environmental Health Professionals. J. E. H. Vol. 38, No. 3. Nov./Dec. 1975. 155-158.

www.ingramcontent.com/pod-product-compliance
Lightning Source LLC
Chambersburg PA
CBHW081908170526
45167CB00007B/3198